CHRONIC MYELOID LEUKEMIA DIET COOKBOOK

Nutrient-Rich Recipes, Foods, And Meal Plans To Boost Immunity, Support Treatment, And Improve Quality Of Life – All You Need To Know

DR. AMARI VALERIE

TABLE OF CONTENTS

BONUS:

7 days meal plan recipes, ingredients, and detailed preparatory guidelines for Chronic Myeloid Leukemia

7 Desserts procedural recipes for Chronic Myeloid Leukemia and guidelines

7 Smoothies procedural recipes for Chronic Myeloid Leukemia and guidelines

DISCLAIMER

The information provided in this book, is for educational and informational purposes only and is not intended as medical advice. The content is not a substitute for professional medical advice, diagnosis, or treatment. Always seek the advice of your physician or other qualified health provider with any questions you may have regarding a medical condition. Never disregard professional medical advice or delay in seeking it because of something you have read in this book.

The dietary suggestions and recipes in this book are based on general guidelines and may not be suitable for everyone. Individual responses to foods can vary, and it is important to consult with a healthcare professional before making any significant changes to your diet.

The author and publisher of this book do not claim to cure or treat any medical condition. The information provided is based on research and personal experience and is intended to help readers make informed decisions about their diet and health.

Furthermore, I the author do not endorse any specific products, brands, treatments, or services that may be mentioned in this book. Any references to products, services, websites, or organizations are provided for informational purposes only and do not constitute an endorsement or recommendation by the author. The inclusion of such references does not imply any association, sponsorship, or affiliation between the author and the referenced entities.

The recipes and dietary suggestions in this book are designed to be safe and healthful. However, readers should use their own discretion and consult with a healthcare professional when necessary, especially if they have allergies, sensitivities, or other dietary restrictions.

By using this book, you acknowledge and agree that the author and publisher shall not be held liable for any loss or damage, including but not limited to special, incidental, consequential, or other damages, resulting from the use of the information and recipes contained in this book.

ABOUT THIS BOOK

This "Chronic Myeloid Leukemia Diet Cookbook" is a critical resource for individuals who are traversing the complexities of Chronic Myeloid Leukemia (CML) and emphasizes the critical role that diet plays in managing this condition. This book commences with a thorough examination of CML, which includes its nature, symptoms, diagnostic procedures, and various phases. It conducts a comprehensive analysis of the variety of available treatment options, emphasizing the critical role that diet plays in improving the efficacy of treatment and the overall management of the disease.

The section on the function of nutrition in CML explores how dietary choices can impact the progression of the disease and the well-being of patients. The benefits of a balanced diet are underscored by the identification of key nutrients that are essential for CML patients. This book does not hesitate to confront the prevalent nutritional obstacles that patients may encounter and offers practical guidance on how to implement the requisite dietary modifications during the treatment phase. This foundation establishes the groundwork for a more thorough investigation into the development of a CML-friendly kitchen, which is furnished with essential tools, nutritious ingredients, and practical advice for safe food handling and meal preparation.

Readers will discover valuable advice on the critical skill of reading and comprehending food labels, which is indispensable for individuals who are managing a chronic illness. This cookbook extends beyond basic recipes by providing structured guidance on the development of nutritious meal plans that are customized to the specific requirements of the individual. It emphasizes the significance of hydration and offers suggestions for efficient meal planning and batch cookery, thereby facilitating the maintenance of patients' dietary regimens.

This book addresses common concerns by offering strategies to manage side effects through diet, address appetite changes, and ensure food safety during treatment. It also evaluates the advantages and disadvantages of supplements, providing answers to frequently inquired questions that patients and caregivers frequently have.

This cookbook provides a diverse selection of protein sources, fruits, vegetables, whole cereals, and healthy lipids in the chapters that are tailored to nutrient-rich foods and immune-boosting recipes. It guides hydration and offers a selection of delectable, immune-boosting recipes for each meal, from breakfast to dessert.

Detailed strategies for various stages of treatment, such as pre-treatment, during treatment, post-treatment, and long-term maintenance, are addressed as part of meal planning. This section is especially beneficial for the creation of meal plans that are tailored to the specific requirements of each patient, thereby guaranteeing that dietary habits adapt to the patient's treatment and recuperation phases.

The management of prevalent side effects through diet is another critical subject that is addressed. Specific foods and dietary modifications are recommended to ameliorate symptoms such as fatigue, vertigo, mouth sores, and digestive discomfort. This book also emphasizes the significance of food safety and provides a list of foods to avoid, such as processed foods, alcohol, caffeine, and high-sodium items.

This section offers practical culinary ideas and techniques to facilitate the preparation of meals. This encompasses concepts for expediting meal preparation, preserving nutrients through culinary methods, augmenting flavors without adding additional calories, and batch cooking. The incorporation of recipes that are suitable for children guarantees that family meals are both nutritious and entertaining.

Also included in this cookbook are specialized sections for desserts and smoothies, as well as a 7-day meal plan that is specifically designed for CML patients, including detailed recipes and preparatory guidelines.

These recipes are intended to be both palatable and nutritious, thereby facilitating patients' compliance with their dietary regimens.

Finally, "Living Well with CML" is a comprehensive approach that incorporates the significance of social support and community resources, as well as physical activity, stress management, and mental health. It promotes the adoption of lifestyle adjustments and regular medical follow-ups to promote long-term health, offering a comprehensive guide for individuals affected by CML.

CHAPTER ONE

Comprehending Chronic Myeloid Leukemia (CML)

Chronic myeloid leukemia (CML) is a form of malignancy that impacts the bone marrow and circulation. It is distinguished by the excessive production of myeloid cells, which are embryonic white blood cells. Fatigue, lethargy, and anemia are symptoms that result from the progressive displacement of healthy cells by these abnormal cells.

Symptoms And Diagnosis

Fatigue, lethargy, fever, nocturnal sweats, and unexplained weight loss are among the symptoms of CML, which can differ from person to person. A blood test is frequently performed to diagnose CML by examining the presence of the Philadelphia chromosome, a genetic abnormality that is frequently associated with the disease. Additionally, elevated white blood cell counts are observed.

Stages Of CML

The chronic, accelerated, and explosion phases are the three periods into which CML is typically divided. The disease progresses slowly during the chronic phase, and many individuals may not experience any discernible symptoms. Nevertheless, it has the potential to progress to the accelerated phase and, in the end, the explosion phase, which is more aggressive and challenging to treat, if left untreated.

Treatment Alternatives For Chronic Myeloid Leukemia

often entails targeted therapy with tyrosine kinase inhibitors (TKIs), which assist in inhibiting the action of the aberrant protein produced by the

Philadelphia chromosome. Chemotherapy, immunotherapy, and stem cell transplantation are additional choices for individuals with advanced disease or those who do not respond well to TKIs.

The Significance Of Diet In The Management Of CML

Although CML cannot be cured by diet alone, it is crucial to maintain a nutritious diet for overall well-being and to support the body during treatment. A diet that is well-balanced and contains a variety of fruits, vegetables, whole cereals, and lean proteins can assist in the maintenance of a healthy weight, the management of adverse effects of treatment such as fatigue and nausea, and the enhancement of the immune system. In addition, it is crucial to maintain proper hydration by consuming an adequate amount of water and reducing the consumption of processed foods, sugary beverages, and alcohol, as these substances can exacerbate fatigue and erode the immune system. Personalized recommendations can be provided by consulting with a registered dietitian, which is determined by the individual's requirements and treatment objectives.

The Involvement Of Nutrition In Chronic Myeloid Leukemia

Nutrition is essential for the management of Chronic Myeloid Leukemia (CML) as it enhances the body's capacity to combat the disease and promotes overall health.

Maintaining a healthy weight, increasing energy levels, and supporting the immune system are all benefits of a well-balanced diet. These factors are crucial for preventing infections and managing the adverse effects of treatment.

The Impact Of Nutrition On Chronic Myeloid Leukemia

The body's capacity to manage CML and its treatments is directly influenced by nutrition. The immune system can be compromised, fatigue can be increased, and adverse effects such as vertigo and gastrointestinal issues can be exacerbated by poor dietary choices. Conversely, a diet that is rich in nutrients can improve the quality of life, strengthen the body, and improve the outcomes of treatment for patients with CML.

Essential Nutrients For Patients With CML

It is advantageous for patients with chronic myeloid leukemia (CML) to consume a diverse array of essential nutrients that promote their health and prosperity. These consist of protein for muscle strength and repair, iron for the prevention of anemia, vitamin C for immune function, and omega-3 fatty acids for the reduction of inflammation. Furthermore, it is imperative to maintain sufficient hydration to mitigate the dehydration that may result from specific medications and treatment adverse effects.

Advantages Of A Well-Balanced Diet

A well-balanced diet offers a variety of advantages to patients with chronic myeloid leukemia (CML), including improved energy levels, more effective management of treatment adverse effects, and improved overall health.

Patients can enhance their nutritional intake and enhance their body's capacity to confront the obstacles of CML and its treatment by incorporating a diverse array of fruits, vegetables, whole cereals, lean proteins, and healthy lipids into their meals.

Common Nutritional Obstacles

Common nutritional challenges that CML patients frequently encounter include nausea, flavor alterations, loss of appetite, and difficulty ingesting. The maintenance of an adequate nutrient intake can be difficult due to these issues, which may lead to weight loss, fatigue, and a reduction in immune function. Nevertheless, these obstacles can be mitigated by employing strategies such as consuming nutrient-dense foods, consuming frequent small meals, and collaborating with a dietitian to guarantee optimal nutrition during treatment.

Dietary Modifications During Treatment

To effectively manage symptoms and adverse effects during treatment for CML, dietary modifications may be required. For instance, a patient who is experiencing nausea may find relief by avoiding oily or spicy foods and instead choosing mild, easily digestible options like rice, toast, or crackers. In the same vein, augmenting fluid intake can mitigate dehydration that is induced by medications such as tyrosine kinase inhibitors. To receive personalized recommendations and support throughout their treatment journey, patients must disclose any dietary concerns to their healthcare team.

CHAPTER TWO

Developing A Kitchen That Is Compliant With A Medical License

A CML-friendly kitchen is achieved by organizing your culinary area to prioritize healthy, nutritious foods while minimizing potential hazards. Begin by organizing your larder and refrigerator by eliminating processed foods that are high in sugar and unhealthy lipids. Substitute them with fruits, vegetables, lean proteins, and whole grains. Designate areas for specific dietary categories to facilitate and optimize meal preparation.

To preserve the quality of fresh produce and remnants and mitigate the risk of contamination, it is advisable to invest in hermetic containers. Finally, to guarantee food safety and prevent cross-contamination, it is crucial to maintain a spotless and well-ventilated kitchen.

Kitchen Gadgets And Tools That Are Essential

Ensuring food safety and nutrition can be achieved by equipping your kitchen with essential tools and devices, which can facilitate meal preparation and cooking. Invest in a high-quality chef's knife for chopping fruits and vegetables, a cutting board made of non-porous material to prevent bacterial development, and a food thermometer to ensure that proteins are cooked to the specified temperature.

Other beneficial devices include non-stick cookware for cooking with minimal oil, a steamer for cooking vegetables without sacrificing nutrients, and a blender for preparing soups and smoothies. In addition to simplifying the process of cooking, these instruments also promote a healthier diet that is beneficial for the management of CML.

Purchasing Nutritious Ingredients In Bulk

Maintaining a balanced diet while managing CML necessitates stocking up on nutritious ingredients. Incorporate a diverse selection of nutrient-dense foods, including whole grains, lean proteins, fruits, and vegetables, into your pantry and refrigerator. Consider quinoa, brown rice, and whole wheat pasta as healthier alternatives to refined cereals. Choose lean meats, such as skinless chicken breast, turkey, and fish, and incorporate plant-based protein sources, such as tofu, lentils, and legumes.

Maintain a diverse intake of vitamins and minerals by maintaining a variety of fresh fruits and vegetables. Opt for a colorful selection. Furthermore, to promote overall health and well-being, it is recommended to accumulate nutritious lipids such as olive oil, almonds, and seeds.

Suggestions For Preparing Meals

Efficient meal preparation is essential for the maintenance of a nutritious diet while managing CML. Begin by devising a weekly meal plan that considers your nutritional requirements and preferences. To expedite the culinary process, prepare ingredients in advance, such as washing and slicing vegetables or marinating meats.

Batch cooking larger quantities of dishes and portioning them out for convenient reheating throughout the week are viable options. Utilize ingredients that are adaptable and can be used in a variety of dishes to reduce waste and save time. Furthermore, to preserve nutrients and enhance the diversity of your meals, consider incorporating various culinary techniques, including grilling, roasting, and steaming.

Safe Food Handling Procedures

It is essential to maintain overall health and prevent infectious illnesses by practicing secure food handling, particularly when managing CML. To mitigate the risk of contamination, it is important to wash your hands thoroughly with detergent and water both before and after handling food. To prevent cross-contamination, it is important to clean cutting surfaces, utensils, and countertops with hot, detergent water after each use.

To prevent the transmission of hazardous microorganisms, it is important to keep raw meats, poultry, and seafood separate from other foods. Use a food thermometer to ensure that foods are cooked to the recommended internal temperature to ensure their safety for consumption. Perishable foods should be refrigerated promptly, and any remains should be stored in hermetic containers to prevent spoilage and preserve their freshness. While managing CML, you can reduce the risk of foodborne illness and promote your overall health by adhering to these food safety guidelines.

CHAPTER THREE

Meal Planning For Patients With Chronic Myeloid Leukemia

Focus on a balanced diet that is abundant in nutrients that are essential for the maintenance of overall health and the support of treatment when planning meals for chronic myeloid leukemia (CML) patients. Incorporate a diverse array of foods from all dietary categories, such as fruits, vegetables, whole grains, lean proteins, and healthy lipids.

Aim for smaller, more frequent meals throughout the day to assist in the regulation of energy levels and the alleviation of digestive discomfort. Consult with a registered dietitian who specializes in oncology nutrition to create customized meal plans that cater to your unique dietary requirements and preferences.

Formulating Well-Balanced Meal Plans

A balanced meal plan for patients with chronic myeloid leukemia (CML) should prioritize nutrient-dense foods while taking into account dietary restrictions and treatment adverse effects. Incorporate a diverse array of vibrant fruits and vegetables to promote immune function and digestion by supplying antioxidants and fiber.

To facilitate muscle mass preservation and recuperation, prioritize lean protein sources, including poultry, fish, tofu, and legumes. For sustained energy and fiber, incorporate whole cereals such as brown rice, quinoa, and whole wheat bread. To enhance overall health and well-being, restrict the consumption of refined foods, sugary treats, and high-fat items.

Incorporating Nutrient-Rich Foods

Nutrient-rich diets are essential for the immune function and overall health of patients with chronic myeloid leukemia (CML). Emphasize the integration of a diverse array of vibrant fruits and vegetables into meals and refreshments to ensure that the body receives the necessary vitamins, minerals, and antioxidants.

For instance, carrots, bell peppers, sweet potatoes, verdant greens, and berries are all examples of this. Select lean protein sources, including chicken, poultry, fish, eggs, and plant-based proteins like tofu and legumes.

Incorporate nutritious lipids from sources such as avocados, nuts, seeds, and olive oil to promote cardiac health and mitigate inflammation.

Suggestions For Batch Cooking And Meal Preparation

Batch cookery and meal preparation can facilitate meal planning and guarantee that CML patients have access to nutritious options at all times. Schedule time each week to prepare ingredients in advance, construct a grocery list, and plan menus. Streamline the culinary process during the hectic weekdays by chopping vegetables, cooking cereals, and portioning out proteins.

Invest in storage containers to facilitate the simple retrieval of prepared ingredients and cooked dishes from the refrigerator or freezer. Throughout the week, it is advisable to prepare versatile staples such as soups, stews, casseroles, and grain bowls that can be personalized with a variety of garnishes and seasonings.

Customizing Meal Plans To Meet The Specific Requirements Of Each Individual

It is imperative to develop personalized meal plans that cater to the distinctive dietary requirements and preferences of patients with chronic myeloid leukemia. When developing meal plans, it is important to take into account factors such as appetite changes, flavor changes, gastrointestinal symptoms, and treatment adverse effects.

Collaborate closely with a registered dietitian to customize dietary recommendations according to the patient's medical history, nutritional status, and treatment objectives. While making modifications to accommodate changing requirements throughout the treatment journey, be receptive to experimenting with new foods and recipes.

To optimize nutritional intake and promote overall well-being, it is essential to periodically assess and adjust meal plans as necessary.

The Significance Of Hydration

CML patients need to maintain hydration levels, manage treatment adverse effects, and support overall health by staying hydrated. It is recommended that you consume an abundance of fluids throughout the day, such as water, medicinal teas, and diluted fruit beverages. Monitor the color and output of urine as a general indicator of hydration status, to achieve pale yellow urine.

Ensure that you have a water bottle readily available to consume regularly, particularly during and after physical activity or exposure to sweltering weather.

Caffeinated beverages and alcohol should be consumed in moderation, as they can lead to dehydration.

Consult with a dietitian for personalized hydration recommendations and be aware of any fluid restrictions recommended by healthcare providers.

CHAPTER FOUR

Frequently Asked Questions And Common Concerns

Many patients are uncertain about the foods they should consume, the foods they should avoid, and how their diet can affect their treatment when it comes to chronic myeloid leukemia (CML).

During treatment, there are several common concerns, including the maintenance of a balanced diet, the management of adverse effects, and the assurance of food safety.

Inquiries regarding specific foods, dietary restrictions, and the function of nutrition in the management of CML symptoms are frequently posed.

Dietary Modifications For The Management Of Side Effects

The management of the adverse effects of CML treatment is significantly influenced by diet. For example, bland, easily digestible foods such as crackers, toast, or fruits may alleviate nausea. Incorporating foods that are high in iron, such as spinach and lean proteins, can increase energy levels and alleviate fatigue.

Furthermore, the management of common side effects such as vertigo and appetite changes can be achieved by maintaining hydration and consuming small, frequent meals throughout the day.

Addressing Changes In Appetite

Treatment adverse effects or the disease itself are frequently the cause of appetite alterations in CML patients. Focus on nutrient-dense foods that are both appealing and simple to consume to address reduced appetite or taste changes. Investigate various flavors and textures to determine which one is most suitable for your preferences. Despite fluctuations in appetite, smoothies, stews, and small, frequent meals can assist in the maintenance of sufficient nutrition.

Food Safety During Treatment

Food safety is of the utmost importance during the treatment of CML, particularly because chemotherapy can impair the immune system. Minimize the risk of contaminated illnesses by practicing proper food handling, storage, and preparation.

Thoroughly wash fruits and vegetables, cook meats to the recommended temperature, and refrain from consuming uncooked seafood and unpasteurized dairy products.

Furthermore, it is advisable to steer clear of foods that pose a greater risk of contamination, such as fresh sprouts and deli meats.

Advantages And Drawbacks Of Supplements

Although supplements may appear to be a convenient method of improving nutrition, they have both advantages and disadvantages for patients with chronic myeloid leukemia. To address specific deficiencies or adverse effects of treatment, certain supplements, such as vitamin D or iron, may be recommended.

Nevertheless, excessive supplementation may result in adverse effects or interactions with medications. Ensure that any new supplements are safe and suitable for your specific requirements by consulting with your healthcare team before taking them.

Nutrient-Rich Foods For Patients With CML

Eating a diet that is abundant in nutrients is essential for the treatment of chronic myeloid leukemia (CML). Consuming a diverse array of foods guarantees that you receive the necessary vitamins and minerals to maintain your overall health and immune system. Maintain a balanced diet by emphasizing lean proteins, fruits, vegetables, whole cereals, and healthy lipids.

Protein Sources: Plant-Based, Fish, And Meat

Protein is indispensable for patients with chronic myeloid leukemia, as it is indispensable for the maintenance of immune function and the repair of cells. Choose lean meats such as poultry, turkey, and fish, which offer high-quality protein without excessive cholesterol. Plant-based alternatives, including pecans, lentils, tofu, and legumes, are also exceptional sources of protein for individuals who adhere to a vegetarian or vegan diet.

Vitamins And Antioxidants Are Present In Fruits And Vegetables.

Vitamins, minerals, and antioxidants are abundant in colorful fruits and vegetables, which aid in the reduction of inflammation and the strengthening of the immune system. To guarantee that you are consuming a diverse array of nutrients to promote your health, incorporate a diversity of options into your diet, such as berries, citrus fruits, leafy vegetables, carrots, and bell peppers.

Fiber-Rich Foods And Whole Grains

In addition to aiding in metabolism, whole cereals are an exceptional source of fiber, which is essential for the maintenance of healthy blood sugar levels. Increase your fiber intake by incorporating whole grains such as brown rice, quinoa, cereals, and whole wheat bread into your meals. Fiber-rich foods also enhance satiety, thereby promoting feelings of fullness and satisfaction following meals.

Omega-3s And Other Beneficial Fats

Heart health is contingent upon the consumption of healthy lipids, which can also mitigate inflammation in the body. To improve your overall health, incorporate omega-3 fatty acid sources such as salmon, sardines, chia seeds, and flaxseeds into your diet. Additionally, avocados, almonds, and olive oil are exceptional sources of healthy lipids that can be incorporated into your diet.

Hydration: The Significance Of Water And Healthy Drinks

It is imperative for all individuals, but particularly for those with CML who are undergoing treatment, to maintain proper hydration.

Consuming an abundance of water facilitates the elimination of impurities from the body and ensures that cells are adequately hydrated and functioning at their best. Aim to consume a minimum of eight glasses of water per day, and diversify your diet by integrating hydrating beverages such as infused water, coconut water, and medicinal teas. Refrain from consuming sugary beverages and excessive caffeine, as they may exacerbate dehydration and may not align with one's overall health objectives.

CHAPTER FIVE

Recipes For Boosting The Immune System

It can be essential to incorporate immune-boosting recipes into your diet to effectively manage chronic myeloid leukemia. Incorporate foods that are high in vitamins, minerals, and antioxidants, such as almonds, seeds, fruits, and vegetables. Consider recipes that include spinach, fruit, and Greek yogurt in smoothies that enhance immunity, or soups that are enriched with turmeric, ginger, and garlic.

Smoothies And Overnight Oats For Breakfast

Begin your day with breakfast options that are both nutritious and simple to prepare, such as overnight oats and smoothies. Combine bananas, spinach, almond milk, and chia seeds to create a smoothie that is rich in nutrients. Alternatively, overnight oats can be made by soaking oats in almond milk and adding garnishes such as diced fruits, nuts, and a drizzle of honey for an extra burst of flavor.

Lunch: Protein-Rich Sandwiches And Salads

For a nutritious lunch, choose salads that are piled high with colorful vegetables, verdant greens, and lean proteins such as tofu or broiled chicken. Engage in an experiment with various dressings, including lemon tahini or balsamic vinaigrette. If you prefer sandwiches, opt for whole-grain bread and load it with protein-rich ingredients such as turkey, avocado, and hummus to enjoy a satisfying meal.

Dinner: Well-balanced meals that include vegetables and lean proteins

Incorporate a variety of vegetables and lean proteins to create nutritious entrees. Pair roasted sweet potatoes and steamed broccoli with salmon that has been seasoned with seasonings and grilled or baked. For a simple and nutritious meal, prepare a stir-fry with tofu, bell peppers, snap peas, and brown rice.

Snacks: Simple And Nutritious Alternatives

To avoid cravings and sustain energy levels throughout the day, it is important to have a variety of nutritious foods available. Consider alternatives such as a sprinkling of mixed nuts and seeds for a satisfying crunch, Greek yogurt with berries, and a dusting of granola, or cut vegetables with hummus.

Desserts: Nutritious And Indulgent Snack

Satisfy your delectable appetite without sacrificing your health by indulging in nutritious desserts. Savor fruit-based delicacies, such as baked apples with cinnamon and a sprinkling of Greek yogurt, or savor a small piece of dark chocolate with sliced strawberries. Experiment with recipes for guilt-free delights, such as chia seed pudding with coconut milk and vanilla extract or avocado chocolate mousse.

Meal Plans For Various Stages Of Treatment

It is essential to customize diet plans to accommodate the different stages of treatment for individuals with Chronic Myeloid Leukemia (CML). To prepare the body for therapy, it is important to prioritize the development of strength through a balanced diet that is abundant in fruits, vegetables, whole cereals, and proteins during pre-treatment.

Manage side effects such as vertigo and loss of appetite by consuming small, frequent meals that are easily digestible, such as soups, smoothies, and wafers, during treatment. After treatment, it is important to prioritize recovery and immune support by consuming nutrient-dense foods such as lean proteins, verdant greens, and citrus fruits. These foods will help to promote healing and increase immunity. To ensure long-term health and well-being, it is important to adopt sustainable dietary practices that encompass a diverse array of foods from all food groups.

Adapting Meal Plans To Meet The Specific Requirements Of Each Individual

Individualized meal plans are indispensable for individuals with CML, as their nutritional requirements may fluctuate contingent upon factors such as age, weight, overall health, and treatment response. Consulting with a registered dietitian can assist in the development of customized meal plans that account for individual nutritional needs and preferences. For instance, certain individuals may require an increase in protein consumption to maintain muscle mass during treatment, while others may require a focus on iron-rich foods to combat anemia. Optimal nutrition and improved treatment outcomes for individuals with CML are achieved by adjusting dietary plans to meet their unique requirements.

CHAPTER SIX

Managing Common Side Effects Through Diet Management

Vomiting And Nausea: Hydration And Gentle Foods

When suffering from nausea and vomiting as a result of Chronic Myeloid Leukemia (CML) or its treatment, it is crucial to prioritize foods that are readily digestible and will not exacerbate symptoms.

Choose neutral, non-greasy foods such as rice, bananas, crostini, and crackers. Eating small, frequent meals can also be beneficial. Maintain hydration by consuming clear fluids such as water, herbal infusions, or electrolyte beverages throughout the day. Eating leisurely and refraining from inhaling strong odors can further alleviate discomfort.

Energy-Boosting Foods: Fatigue

Fatigue is a prevalent adverse effect of CML and its treatments; however, it is possible to mitigate this by altering one's diet. Incorporate energy-boosting foods, such as complex carbohydrates (whole cereals, legumes), lean proteins (chicken, fish, tofu), and healthy lipids (avocado, nuts, olive oil), into your meals. Strive to consume nutritious nibbles and meals that are well-balanced to sustain consistent energy levels throughout the day. Furthermore, it is possible to prevent energy declines by maintaining hydration and restricting caffeine and sugary foods.

Mouth Sores And Difficulty Swallowing: Soft And Smooth Foods

For those with CML, dining can be a difficult task due to mouth sores and difficulty ingesting. Focus on soft and smooth foods that are easier to digest and ingest to alleviate discomfort.

The following are some examples: yogurt, pureed potatoes, smoothies, and stews. Refrain from consuming foods that are acidic, peppery, or have a rough texture, as they may exacerbate the itchiness of ulcers. Additionally, by drinking through a tiny spoon or using a straw, it is possible to circumvent sore areas in the mouth.

Weight Fluctuations: Strategies For Managing Weight Gain And Loss

Weight fluctuations, including both weight reduction and weight gain, may manifest during the treatment of CML. Focus on calorie-dense foods, such as almonds, nut butter, cheese, and preserved fruits, for individuals who are experiencing weight loss to increase their intake.

It is also possible to maintain muscle mass by incorporating protein-rich foods and healthful lipids.

However, if weight gain is a concern, it is important to prioritize portion control and emphasize whole, nutrient-dense foods, while limiting high-calorie, processed options. Regular physical activity can also assist in the pursuit of weight management objectives.

Digestive Disorders: Probiotics And Fiber

During the treatment of CML, digestive issues such as diarrhea or constipation may develop. By fostering regular bowel movements, constipation can be alleviated by increasing fiber intake through fruits, vegetables, whole cereals, and legumes.

Nevertheless, individuals who are experiencing diarrhea may find it advantageous to temporarily decrease their fiber intake and concentrate on simple-to-digest foods such as applesauce, pears, and white rice.

Healthy intestinal flora can be restored and digestion can be enhanced by consuming probiotic-rich foods such as yogurt and kefir.

To effectively manage digestive symptoms, it is crucial to heed your body and modify your diet as necessary.

CHAPTER SEVEN

Foods To Avoid And The Reasons For Their Avoidance

In the management of chronic myeloid leukemia (CML), it is essential to refrain from consuming specific foods that may exacerbate symptoms or obstruct treatment. Cardiovascular health is a concern for CML patients, as certain treatments may have potential cardiovascular adverse effects. High-fat dairy products, such as whole milk and cheese, can increase cholesterol levels.

In the same vein, it is advisable to refrain from consuming raw or undercooked meats and seafood to mitigate the risk of contaminated illnesses. These illnesses can be particularly hazardous for individuals with compromised immune systems, a condition that is prevalent among CML patients who are undergoing treatment.

Sugary And Processed Foods

Processed foods, including packaged munchies, tinned soups, and fast food, frequently contain high levels of sodium, preservatives, and artificial additives, which can be detrimental to overall health and contribute to inflammation. Furthermore, the consumption of sugary foods and beverages, such as soda, chocolates, and pastries, can result in blood sugar surges, which may exacerbate insulin resistance and elevate the risk of diabetes. This condition is something that CML patients must manage in conjunction with their leukemia treatment.

Caffeine And Alcohol

Individuals with CML should either limit or abstain from alcohol consumption, as it can exacerbate the adverse effects of certain medications used to treat the disease and interfere with liver function. In the same vein, while moderate caffeine consumption is generally regarded as safe for the majority of individuals, excessive caffeine consumption can result in dehydration and disrupt sleep patterns, both of which can have a detrimental effect on overall well-being and immune function. These are critical factors to consider for individuals who are managing CML.

Foods That Are High In Sodium

Foods that are high in sodium, such as processed meats, canned soups, and salty munchies, should be restricted in a CML diet. This is because they have the potential to increase blood pressure and contribute to fluid retention, which may exacerbate symptoms such as swelling and edema that are frequently associated with this condition. Instead, consuming fresh, whole foods and enhancing the flavor of dishes with seasonings and spices can help reduce sodium intake while simultaneously enhancing the nutritional value and flavor of meals.

Herbal Products And Specific Supplements

Although herbal products and supplements are frequently advertised as natural remedies for a variety of health conditions, including cancer, individuals with CML must exercise caution when utilizing them. Certain supplements, including vitamin E and specific herbal remedies like ginseng and echinacea, may interact with CML medications or impede the body's ability to metabolize them, potentially resulting in their ineffectiveness or severe adverse effects.

It is imperative to consult with a healthcare provider before initiating any new supplement regimen to guarantee the safety and efficacy of CML management.

Food Safety: Preventing Contaminants

It is of the utmost importance to ensure the safety of food for individuals with CML, as their immune systems may be compromised as a result of the disease or its treatment. This requires the thorough rinsing of fruits and vegetables before consumption, the cooking of meats and seafood to their recommended internal temperatures to eliminate harmful bacteria, and the avoidance of unpasteurized dairy products and undercooked eggs, which can harbor pathogens such as Salmonella and E. E. coli.

Furthermore, proper food storage and handling techniques can mitigate the risk of contaminated illnesses and prevent cross-contamination, which can be especially hazardous for those with compromised immune systems.

Techniques And Advice For Cooking

It is essential to prioritize culinary methods that preserve nutrients and reduce the consumption of superfluous lipids and sugars when preparing food for chronic myeloid leukemia (CML). Select cooking methods that require minimal oil, such as steaming, roasting, barbecuing, or stir-frying. Refrain from deep-frying or utilizing an excessive quantity of butter or cream. Furthermore, to enhance the flavor of the dish without resorting to sodium or sugar, contemplate the use of citrus juices, seasonings, and herbs.

Meal Preparation Ideas That Are Quick And Simple

When preparing meals for CML, efficiency is paramount. Plan your meals and choose recipes that necessitate minimal preparation. Consider batch-cooking cereals such as brown rice or quinoa, pre-chopping vegetables, and marinating proteins for subsequent rapid preparation. Utilize kitchen appliances such as pressure cookers or slow cookers to prepare nutritious dishes promptly.

Cooking To Preserve Nutrients

Focus on culinary methods that preserve nutrients to guarantee that you are obtaining the maximum amount of those nutrients from your food. This can be achieved by steaming, microwaving, or gently sautéing vegetables to preserve their vitamins and minerals. To preserve the protein content of flesh, it is important to avoid overcooking it. Maximize your nutrient intake by incorporating a diverse array of vibrant fruits and vegetables into your meals.

Flavor Enhancements Without Additional Calories

With the appropriate ingredients, it is possible to improve the flavor of your meals without introducing additional calories. To enhance the profundity and complexity of your dishes, experiment with herbs, seasonings, vinegar, and citrus juices. Basil, cilantro, and parsley are examples of fresh herbs that can enhance the flavor of salads, soups, and marinades without adding additional calories. Adding richness without excess fat is also possible by substituting heavier sauces with flavorful broths or stocks.

Convenient Batch Cooking And Freezing

When managing CML, batch preparing and freezing portions can be a savior. Prepare large quantities of soups, stews, or casseroles that can be simply divided into individual portions and frozen for future use. Invest in freezer-safe containers or sacks to ensure that meals are stored efficiently. To monitor the condition of each object, it is important to label and date it. This approach guarantees that you always have nutritious, prepared alternatives at your disposal, thereby reducing the likelihood of selecting less nutritious convenience foods.

Recipes For Family Meals That Are Suitable For Children

It is crucial to identify recipes that are both nutritious and appealing to young palates when catering to a family, including children. Incorporate common ingredients in innovative ways, such as merging them into smoothies or incorporating them into homemade pizzas. Allow children to participate in the culinary process by allowing them to assist with basic duties such as stirring, measuring ingredients, or assembling wraps or sandwiches. By involving them in the preparation of meals, you can not only promote healthy eating habits from a young age but also enhance the overall enjoyment of mealtime for the entire family.

CHAPTER EIGHT

Seven-Day Meal Plan, Recipes, Ingredients, And Detailed Preparatory Guidelines For Chronic Myeloid Leukemia

Significant Factors To Take Into Account

• Foods that reduce inflammation: Consume an abundance of fruits, vegetables, whole cereals, and lean proteins.

• Refrain from consuming processed foods: Reduce the consumption of sugary and processed foods.

• Hydration: Maintain proper hydration by consuming water and fresh beverages.

• Small, frequent meals: To regulate appetite and prevent fatigue.

THE FIRST DAY

BREAKFAST

Oatmeal with Berries and Nuts

INGREDIENTS:

• One cup of rolled oats

• Two glasses of almond milk or water

• 1/2 cup of assorted berries (strawberries, blueberries)

• One tablespoon of chia seeds

• 1 tablespoon of pulverized nuts (walnuts, almonds)

• One teaspoon of honey (optional)

PREPARATION:

1. In a kettle, bring the water or almond milk to a boil.

2. Reduce the heat and incorporate grains. Stir occasionally while cooking for 5-7 minutes.

3. Add berries, chia seeds, almonds, and honey to the top.

Quinoa and Vegetable Salad

INGREDIENTS:

• One cup of prepared quinoa

• Half a cup of cherry tomatoes

• Diced cucumber, 1/2

• One-quarter of a finely sliced red onion

• Crumbled 1/4 cup of feta cheese

• Two tablespoons of olive oil

• One tablespoon of lemon juice

• Salt and pepper to flavor

PREPARATION:

1. In a sizable basin, combine feta, tomatoes, cucumber, onion, and quinoa.

2. Combine olive oil, lemon juice, salt, and pepper in a small basin.

3. Combine the salad by pouring the vinaigrette over it and tossing it.

Dinner

Steamed Vegetables with Baked Salmon

INGREDIENTS:

• One salmon tenderloin

• One tablespoon of olive oil

• Salt and pepper to flavor

• One lemon, sliced

• A variety of mixed vegetables, including broccoli, carrots, and green beans

PREPARATION:

1. Preheat the oven to 375°F (190°C).

2. Place the salmon on a baking sheet, drizzle with olive oil, and season with salt and pepper.

3. Place lemon segments on top of the salmon.

4. Bake for 20-25 minutes.

5. Steam vegetables until they are soft.

Snack

Greek yogurt with honey and walnuts

INGREDIENTS:

• One cup of Greek yogurt

• One teaspoon of honey

• One tablespoon of pulverized walnuts

PREPARATION:

1. Combine hazelnuts and honey in the yogurt.

Juice

Green Detox Juice

INGREDIENTS:

• One cup of spinach

• One cucumber

• Two stalks of celery

• One apple

• Juice from one lemon

• A one-inch slice of ginger

PREPARATION:

1. All ingredients should be blended until they are homogeneous. If desirable, strain the mixture.

THE SECOND DAY

Breakfast

Smoothie Bowl

INGREDIENTS:

• One banana

• 1/2 cup of thawed fruit

• One-half cup of almond milk

• One tablespoon of almond butter

• One tablespoon of chia seeds

• Granola for garnishing

PREPARATION:

1. Blend almond butter, almond milk, banana, and berries until they are completely smooth.

2. Transfer the mixture to a vessel and garnish with granola and chia seeds.

Lentil Soup

INGREDIENTS:

- One cup of drained legumes

- One diced onion

- Two carrots, sliced

- Two sliced celery stalks

- Three minced garlic cloves

- Six pints of vegetable broth

- One can of diced tomatoes

- 1 teaspoon of spice

- Salt and pepper to flavor

PREPARATION:

1. Sauté onion, carrots, celery, and garlic in a substantial saucepan until they are tender.

2. Combine lentils, broth, tomatoes, cumin, salt, and pepper.

3. Bring the mixture to a boil, and then allow it to simmer for 30 to 40 minutes.

Dinner

Grilled chicken with asparagus and quinoa

INGREDIENTS:

• One chicken breast

• One cup of prepared quinoa

• One bundle of asparagus, trimmed

• Two tablespoons of olive oil

• Salt and pepper to flavor

• Juice from one lemon

PREPARATION:

1. Sprinkle lemon juice, salt, and pepper over the chicken.

2. Grill poultry until it is completely cooked.

3. Grill asparagus until it is tender, then toss it with olive oil, salt, and pepper.

4. Serve poultry with asparagus and quinoa.

Snack

Apple Slices with Almond Butter

INGREDIENTS:

• One apple, cut

• Two tablespoons of almond butter

PREPARATION:

1. Spread almond butter over apple slices.

Juice

Apple-carrot-ginger juice

INGREDIENTS:

• Four carrots

• Two apples

• A one-inch slice of ginger

PREPARATION:

1. Combine all ingredients for juicing.

THIRD DAY

Breakfast

Avocado Toast with Eggs

INGREDIENTS:

• One piece of whole-grain bread

• Mashed half of an avocado

• Two eggs

• Red pepper flakes, salt, and pepper to flavor

PREPARATION:

1. Toast the bread.

2. Apply pureed avocado to toast.

3. Prepare eggs according to your preference, whether you prefer them poached, scrambled, or otherwise.

4. Season avocado crostini and place eggs on it.

Lunchtime

Chickpea and Spinach Stew

INGREDIENTS:

• One can of legumes, drained and rinsed

• One diced onion

• Two minced garlic cloves

- Two cups of spinach

- One can of diced tomatoes

- 1 teaspoon of spice

- Salt and pepper to flavor

PREPARATION:

1. Sauté garlic and onion until they are tender.

2. Combine tomatoes, cumin, salt, and pepper with the legumes.

3. Allow the mixture to simmer for 20 minutes.

4. Add spinach and simmer until it is wilted.

Dinner

Stuffed bell peppers

INGREDIENTS:

- Four bell peppers, with the stems removed and the seeds removed

• One cup of brown rice that has been prepared

• 1/2 pound of ground turkey

• One diced onion

• Two minced garlic cloves

• One can of diced tomatoes

• One teaspoon of Italian seasoning

• Salt and pepper to flavor

PREPARATION:

1. Turn the oven on to 375°F, or 190°C.

2. First, sauté the onion and garlic. Subsequently, incorporate minced turkey and cook until it is golden brown.

3. Add rice, tomatoes, seasoning, salt, and pepper. Stir to combine.

4. Fill bell peppers with the mixture.

5. Place in a baking dish and bake for 30-35 minutes.

Snack

Hummus and vegetable sticks

INGREDIENTS:

• One cup of hummus

• A variety of vegetable spears, including carrots, celery, and bell peppers

PREPARATION:

1. Dip vegetable skewers in hummus.

Juice

Beetroot and Berry Juice

INGREDIENTS:

• Two beets, peeled

• One single cup of assorted fruit

• One apple

• Juice from one lemon

PREPARATION:

1. Combine all ingredients for juicing.

THE FOURTH DAY

Breakfast

Chia Pudding

INGREDIENTS:

• 1/4 cup of chia seeds

• One cup of almond milk

• 1 teaspoon of vanilla extract

• One tablespoon of maple syrup

• Fresh citrus for garnish

PREPARATION:

1. Combine almond milk, maple syrup, vanilla, and chia seeds.

2. Place in the refrigerator for the night.

3. Add some fresh fruit as a garnish before serving.

Lunchtime

Chicken Breast Stuffed with Spinach and Feta

INGREDIENTS

• One chicken breast

• 1 cup of wilted spinach

• Crumbled 1/4 cup of feta cheese

• One tablespoon of olive oil

• Salt and pepper to flavor

PREPARATION:

1. Preheat the oven to 375°F (190°C).

2. Create a pocket in the chicken breast.

3. Fill with feta and spinach.

4. Season the meat with salt and pepper, and then sear it in a pan with olive oil until it is browned.

5. Bake in the oven for twenty to twenty-five minutes.

Dinner

Stir-fry of Vegetables with Tofu

INGREDIENTS:

• One block of firm tofu, cubed

• One cup of broccoli florets

• One sliced bell pepper

• One sliced carrot

• One zucchini, sliced

• Two tablespoons of soy sauce

• One tablespoon of olive oil

• 1 teaspoon of minced ginger

• 1 teaspoon of minced garlic

PREPARATION:

1. Heat oil in a pan and sauté tofu until it turns golden.

2. Remove tofu and add garlic, ginger, and vegetables to the pan.

3. Stir-fry for 5-7 minutes, then add soy sauce.

4. Return tofu to the pan and mix well.

Mixed Nuts and Dried Fruit

INGREDIENTS:

• 1/4 cup mixed nuts

• 1/4 cup dried fruit

PREPARATION:

1. Mix the dried fruit with the nuts.

Pineapple and Mint Juice

INGREDIENTS:

• One cup of pineapple slices

• A handful of fresh mint leaves

• 1 lime, juiced

PREPARATION:

1. Combine all ingredients for juicing.

DAY FIVE

Breakfast

Fruit and Yogurt Parfait

INGREDIENTS:

• One cup of Greek yogurt

• 1/2 cup granola

• One single cup of assorted fruit

• One tablespoon of honey

PREPARATION:

1. Arrange yogurt, granola, and berries in a glass.

2. Use honey to drizzle.

Turkey and Avocado Wrap

INGREDIENTS:

- 1 whole-grain tortilla

- 3 slices turkey breast

- One half of an avocado, divided

- 1/4 cup shredded lettuce

- 1 tomato, sliced

- 1 tbsp hummus

PREPARATION:

1. Apply hummus to the tortilla.

2. Layer turkey, avocado, lettuce, and tomato.

3. Fold in half and roll up.

Shrimp and Vegetable Skewers

INGREDIENTS:

• 1 lb shrimp, peeled and deveined

• 1 bell pepper, cut into chunks

• One zucchini, sliced

• 1 red onion, cut into chunks

• Two tablespoons of olive oil

• One tablespoon of lemon juice

• Salt and pepper to flavor

PREPARATION:

1. Preheat the grill to medium-high fire.

2. Thread shrimp and vegetables onto skewers.

3. Drizzle with olive oil, lemon juice, salt, and pepper.

4. Grill each side for two to three minutes.

Snack

Edamame

INGREDIENTS:

• 1 cup edamame, cooked

• Salt to flavor

PREPARATION:

1. Sprinkle salt over cooked edamame.

Juice

Orange and Carrot Juice

INGREDIENTS:

• 3 oranges, peeled

• Four carrots

PREPARATION:

1. Combine all ingredients for juicing.

SIXTH DAY

Breakfast

Whole Grain Pancakes with Blueberries

INGREDIENTS:

• 1 cup whole-grain flour

• 1 tbsp baking powder

• One cup of almond milk

• One egg

• One tablespoon of honey

• One-half cup of blueberries

PREPARATION:

1. Mix flour and baking powder in a bowl.

2. In another bowl, mix milk, egg, and honey.

3. Mix the ingredients, wet and dry.

4. Incorporate blueberries by folding.

5. Pancakes should be griddle-cooked till golden brown.

Lunchtime

Mixed Bean Salad

INGREDIENTS:

• 1 can mixed beans, drained and rinsed

• 1/2 red bell pepper, diced

• 1/2 green bell pepper, diced

• One-quarter of a finely sliced red onion

• Two tablespoons of olive oil

• One tablespoon of lemon juice

• Salt and pepper to flavor

PREPARATION:

1. Combine beans, peppers, and onion in a bowl.

2. Mix olive oil, lemon juice, salt, and pepper.

3. Combine the salad by pouring the vinaigrette over it and tossing it.

Dinner

Chicken and Vegetable Stir-Fry

INGREDIENTS:

• 1 chicken breast, sliced

• One cup of broccoli florets

• One sliced bell pepper

- One sliced carrot

- 1 onion, sliced

- Two tablespoons of soy sauce

- One tablespoon of olive oil

- 1 teaspoon of minced garlic

- 1 teaspoon of minced ginger

PREPARATION:

1. Heat oil in a pan and cook chicken until browned.

2. Remove chicken and add garlic, ginger, and vegetables.

3. Stir-fry for 5-7 minutes, then add soy sauce and chicken.

4. Mix well and cook for another 2-3 minutes.

INGREDIENTS:

- 2 rice cakes

- 2 tbsp peanut butter

- 1 banana, sliced

PREPARATION:

1. Spread peanut butter on rice cakes.

2. Top with banana slices.

Juice

Mango and Spinach Smoothie

INGREDIENTS:

- One cup of spinach

- 1 mango, peeled and chopped

- One banana

- One cup of coconut water

PREPARATION:

1. All ingredients should be blended until they are homogeneous.

SEVENTH DAY

Breakfast

Scrambled Tofu with Spinach and Tomatoes

INGREDIENTS:

- 1 block of firm tofu, crumbled

- One cup of spinach

- Half a cup of cherry tomatoes

- 1 tsp turmeric

- 1 tsp olive oil

• Salt and pepper to flavor

PREPARATION:

1. Heat oil in a pan and add tofu.

2. Sprinkle turmeric, salt, and pepper.

3. Add spinach and tomatoes.

4. Cook until vegetables are tender and tofu is heated through.

Lunchtime

Butternut squash soup

INGREDIENTS:

• 1 butternut squash, peeled and cubed

• One diced onion

• Two minced garlic cloves

• 4 cups vegetable broth

• One tablespoon of olive oil

• Salt and pepper to flavor

PREPARATION:

1. Sauté onion and garlic in olive oil until soft.

2. Add squash and broth.

3. Bring to a boil, then simmer until squash is tender.

4. Blend until smooth and season with salt and pepper.

Dinner

Turkey Meatballs with Zucchini Noodles

INGREDIENTS:

• One pound of minced turkey

• 1/4 cup of breadcrumbs

• One egg

• 1/4 cup parmesan cheese, grated

• 2 zucchinis, spiralized

• 1 cup marinara sauce

• One tablespoon of olive oil

• Salt and pepper to flavor

PREPARATION:

1. Preheat the oven to 375°F (190°C).

2. Mix turkey, breadcrumbs, egg, parmesan, salt, and pepper.

3. Shape the mixture into meatballs and arrange them on a baking sheet.

4. Bake for 20-25 minutes.

5. Heat olive oil in a pan and sauté zucchini noodles until tender.

6. Serve meatballs over zucchini noodles with marinara sauce.

Cottage Cheese with Pineapple

INGREDIENTS:

• 1 cup cottage cheese

• 1/2 cup of pineapple segments

PREPARATION:

1. Mix pineapple chunks into cottage cheese.

Watermelon and Cucumber Juice

INGREDIENTS:

• 2 cups watermelon chunks

• One cucumber

PREPARATION:

1. Combine all ingredients for juicing.

This meal plan provides balanced, nutrient-rich meals to support the health and well-being of individuals with Chronic Myeloid Leukemia. Remember to consult with a healthcare provider or a dietitian for personalized advice.

CHAPTER NINE

7 Procedural Dessert Recipes For Chronic Myeloid Leukemia And Guidelines

The adverse effects of treatment frequently present dietary challenges for patients with Chronic Myeloid Leukemia (CML). Proper nutrition is essential for the maintenance of vitality and the enhancement of the immune system. Seven dessert recipes that are specifically designed for CML patients, with an emphasis on nutrient density, reduced sugar content, and simple assimilation, are provided below.

Dessert Guidelines:

1. Low Sugar: Inflammation and other health issues can be exacerbated by a high-sugar diet. Make use of natural sweeteners, such as stevia, maple syrup, or honey.

2. High Fiber: Fiber is essential for the maintenance of healthy blood sugar levels and aids in digestion. Incorporate fruits, vegetables, and whole grains.

3. Healthy Fats: To promote overall health and provide energy, incorporate sources of healthy fats, including avocados, almonds, and seeds.

4. Ingredients Rich in Antioxidants: Berries, dark chocolate, and almonds are included to combat oxidative stress.

5. Ingredients Rich in Probiotics: Yogurt is an example of an ingredient that can assist in the preservation of digestive health, which is frequently impaired during cancer treatment.

6. Hydration: Incorporate ingredients with a high water content to aid in maintaining hydration.

7. Protein: Ensure that there is an adequate amount of protein to support muscle mass and repair tissues.

• Two cups of almond milk • Half a cup of chia seeds • One cup of a blend of fruit, such as blueberries, strawberries, and raspberries • Two tablespoons of maple syrup or honey • One teaspoon of vanilla extract

PROCESS:

1. In a basin, combine almond milk, chia seeds, honey, and vanilla extract.

2. Ensure that the chia seeds are evenly distributed by stirring the mixture thoroughly.

3. Allow the mixture to settle for five minutes before stirring it once more to prevent clotting.

4. Cover and refrigerate for a minimum of four hours or overnight.

5. Before serving, garnish with a variety of berries.

Advantages: Rich in omega-3 fatty acids, antioxidants, and fiber.

2. AVOCADO CHOCOLATE MOUSSE

The following are the components of the recipe: • Two mature avocados • 1/4 cup of unsweetened cocoa powder • 1/4 cup of maple syrup or honey • 1/4 cup of almond milk • One teaspoon of vanilla extract

PROCEDURES:

1. Combine avocados, cocoa powder, honey, almond milk, and vanilla extract in a blender until the mixture is homogeneous.

2. After 30 minutes of chilling, serve.

Advantages: Offers antioxidants, fiber, and healthful lipids.

3. YOGURT PARFAIT INGREDIENTS: • TWO CONTAINERS OF GREEK YOGURT

• One cup of low-sugar granola • One cup of mixed fruit • Two teaspoons of honey

PROCEDURES:

1. In a glass or basin, arrange yogurt, granola, and berries in a layering fashion.

2. Treat the afflicted region with honey.

Advantages: High in antioxidants, probiotics, and protein.

4. OATMEAL COOKIES INGREDIENTS:

• One cup of rolled oats • 1/2 cup of whole wheat flour • 1/2 cup of pureed banana • 1/4 cup of honey • 1/4 cup of raisins • 1 teaspoon of cinnamon • 1 teaspoon of baking powder

PROCEDURES:

1. Set the oven's temperature to 175°C/350°F.

2. Combine all ingredients in a dish.

3. Place tablespoon-sized disks onto a baking sheet.

4. Bake for 10-12 minutes or until the surface is a deep golden brown.

Advantages: Rich in fiber and minimal in refined sugar.

5. APPLE CINNAMON QUINOA INGREDIENTS:

• One cup of quinoa that has been prepared • One apple that has been minced • One teaspoon of cinnamon • One tablespoon of honey • 1/4 cup of chopped almonds (optional)

PROCEDURES:

1. Combine cooked quinoa with honey, cinnamon, and diced apple.

2. If preferred, sprinkle with almonds.

Advantages: Rich in antioxidants, fiber, and protein.

6. FROZEN BANANA BITES INGREDIENTS:

• Two bananas • Half a cup of dark chocolate pieces

• 1/4 cup of pulverized almonds or desiccated coconut • 1 tablespoon of coconut oil

PROCEDURES:

1. Cut bananas into bite-sized segments.

2. Combine coconut oil and dark chocolate morsels to melt.

3. Dip the banana pieces into the molten chocolate and then coat them with almonds or coconut.

4. Allow the mixture to remain in the freezer for a minimum of one hour.

Advantages: Offers antioxidants, potassium, and healthful lipids.

7. PUMPKIN SMOOTHIE INGREDIENTS:

• One banana • One cup of pumpkin puree

• One cup of almond milk • One tablespoon of honey • One teaspoon of pumpkin pie spice

PROCEDURES:

1. The ingredients should be incorporated until they are homogeneous.

2. Before serving, chill the meal.

Advantages: High in antioxidants, fiber, and vitamins A and C.

In summary, these confection recipes provide a harmonious combination of nutrients that can be used to promote the health and well-being of patients with chronic myeloid leukemia.

These desserts can offer both nutrition and solace by incorporating ingredients that are high in protein and healthy fats, high in antioxidants, and simple to metabolize.

It is imperative to seek the advice of a healthcare provider or a dietitian to customize dietary choices to meet the unique health requirements and treatment plans of each individual.

CHAPTER TEN

7 Smoothies Procedural Recipes That Are Appropriate For Individuals With Chronic Myeloid Leukemia, As Well As Guidelines

Chronic myeloid leukemia (CML) is a form of malignancy that impacts the bone marrow and circulation. Although medication and occasionally other medical interventions are the primary treatment, maintaining a nutritious diet can contribute to overall health and well-being. Smoothies are an exceptional method for ingesting essential nutrients.

Seven smoothies that are specifically designed for CML patients are presented below. These smoothies are intended to enhance energy levels, increase immunity, and promote overall health.

Ingredients: • One cup of spinach • Half a cup of kale • One cored and sliced green apple • Half a cucumber • Half a lemon, juiced • A one-inch slice of ginger • One cup of water or coconut water

PROCEDURES:

1. Thoroughly rinse all greens.

2. Combine spinach, kale, green apple, cucumber, lemon juice, and ginger in a blender.

3. Add the water or coconut water.

4. Continue to blend the mixture until it is consistent.

5. For optimal nutrient retention, serve immediately.

Benefits: This smoothie is abundant in antioxidants, folate, and vitamins A, C, and K, which can aid in the detoxification process and strengthen the immune system.

Ingredients: • One banana • One-half cup of blueberries • Half a cup of hulled strawberries • Half a cup of raspberries

• One tablespoon of chia seeds • One cup of purified almond milk

PROCEDURES:

1. Thoroughly rinse all of the berries.

2. Combine almond milk, chia seeds, banana, and berries in a Vitamix.

3. Continue to blend the mixture until it is consistent.

4. Transfer the beverage to a glass and relish it.

Benefits: Antioxidants are essential for the body's defense against oxidative stress and inflammation. Berries are abundant in these compounds.

3. TROPICAL TURMERIC SMOOTHIE

Ingredients: • One cup of pineapple slices • Half a mango, peeled and chopped • 1/2 teaspoon of turmeric powder • 1/2 teaspoon of cinnamon • 1/4 teaspoon of black pepper • One cup of coconut milk

PROCEDURES:

1. Combine coconut milk, turmeric, cinnamon, black pepper, pineapple, and mango in a blender.

2. Blend the mixture until it is creamy and velvety.

3. Chill the dish before serving.

Benefits: This smoothie can assist in the maintenance of the immune system by combining the potent anti-inflammatory properties of turmeric with the vitamin C found in pineapple and mango.

4. PROTEIN-PACKED SMOOTHIE

Ingredients: • One-half cup of Greek yogurt

• One banana

• 2 teaspoons of peanut butter • 1 tablespoon of honey • 1 cup of milk (dairy or plant-based) • 1 tablespoon of flaxseeds

PROCEDURES:

1. Combine Greek yogurt, banana, peanut butter, honey, milk, and flaxseeds in a blender.

2. Continue to blend the mixture until it is consistent.

3. Enjoy immediately.

Benefits: This smoothie is an excellent source of protein, nutritious lipids, and fiber, all of which are crucial for the preservation of overall energy levels and muscle mass.

5. AVOCADO SPINACH SMOOTHIE

Ingredients: • 1 mature avocado • 1 cup of spinach • 1 cored and sliced green apple • 1/2 lime, juiced • 1 cup of coconut water

PROCEDURES:

1. Remove the avocado interior and place it in the blender.

2. Incorporate spinach, green apple, lime juice, and coconut water.

3. Continue to blend the mixture until it is consistent.

4. Serve immediately.

Benefits: Avocado is abundant in healthful fats and minerals, while spinach and green apples offer essential nutrients and antioxidants.

6. BEETROOT BOOST SMOOTHIE

Ingredients: • 1 small beetroot, peeled and chopped • 1 carrot, peeled and chopped • 1 apple, cored and sliced • A one-inch slice of ginger • 1 cup of orange juice

PROCEDURES:

1. Combine orange juice, apple, ginger, beetroot, and carrot in a blender.

2. Continue to blend the mixture until it is consistent.

3. If desirable, strain the mixture and serve it cool.

Benefit: Beetroot is highly effective in enhancing blood flow and oxygenation, while ginger and citrus juice contribute immune-boosting and anti-inflammatory properties.

7. BREAKFAST SMOOTHIE WITH OATMEAL

Ingredients:

• One banana • One-half cup of Greek yogurt • 1/2 cup of rolled cereals

• One tablespoon of honey • One cup of almond milk • Half a teaspoon of cinnamon

PROCEDURES:

1. Finely grind rolled oats by blending them.

2. Incorporate a banana, Greek yogurt, honey, almond milk, and cinnamon into the blender.

3. Continue to blend the mixture until it is consistent.

4. Serve promptly as a nutritious breakfast option.

Benefits: This smoothie is an excellent source of protein and fiber, which will help you remain energized and satisfied throughout the morning.

CML Patients' Recommendations

1. Emphasize Whole Foods: Emphasize the consumption of fresh fruits, vegetables, whole cereals, lean proteins, and healthy lipids.

2. Hydration: Ensure that you consume an adequate amount of fluids, predominantly through water, herbal beverages, and nutrient-rich smoothies.

3. Balanced Diet: Consume a variety of micronutrients (vitamins and minerals) and macronutrients (carbohydrates, proteins, and lipids).

4. Restrict the Consumption of Processed Foods: Prevent the consumption of processed foods that are high in sugar, sodium, and unhealthy lipids.

5. Monitor Caloric Intake: Maintain energy levels and body weight by ensuring an adequate caloric intake, while avoiding excessive calories.

6. Consult with Healthcare Providers: Before implementing substantial dietary modifications, it is imperative to seek the advice of a healthcare provider or nutritionist.

These beverages, which are abundant in essential nutrients, can contribute to the maintenance of overall health and enhance the treatment regimen for CML. The immune system can be strengthened, energy levels can be improved, and overall well-being can be promoted by consuming these nutrient-dense beverages regularly.

CHAPTER ELEVEN

Living A Healthy Life With CML

The adoption of a balanced lifestyle that promotes overall health and well-being is essential for living well with Chronic Myeloid Leukemia (CML). This encompasses the following: adhering to medical follow-ups, seeking social support, managing tension effectively, remaining physically active, and maintaining a nutritious diet. Individuals with CML can enhance their health outcomes and quality of life by incorporating these aspects into their daily routines.

Physical Activity Integration

Individuals with CML need to integrate regular physical activity into their daily routines. Exercise not only enhances physical strength and endurance but also elevates mood and alleviates tension. Walking, swimming, or practicing yoga are straightforward exercises that may prove advantageous. It is imperative to commence with a low level of intensity and progressively increase it, while also heeding the signals of your body and seeking guidance from healthcare providers for personalized recommendations.

Mental Health And Stress Management

It is essential for individuals with CML to effectively manage tension to preserve their overall well-being. Stress can be mitigated through mindfulness, meditation, and deep breathing exercises. Furthermore, valuable emotional support can be obtained by participating in pleasurable activities, spending time with loved ones, and seeking assistance from mental health professionals or support groups.

Community Resources And Social Support

Individuals with CML can derive substantial advantages from seeking social support and utilizing community resources. Connecting with others who comprehend the obstacles of living with CML is facilitated by participating in support groups or online forums, which fosters a sense of belonging and comprehension. Furthermore, practical support and information can be obtained by tapping into community resources, including financial assistance programs, educational seminars, or counseling services.

Regular Health Examinations

Effective management of CML necessitates consistent medical follow-ups. Healthcare providers can promptly address any emergent concerns, assess the efficacy of treatment, and monitor the progression of the disease during these appointments. To optimize outcomes and guarantee early intervention if necessary, it is essential to attend all scheduled appointments, communicate openly with healthcare providers, and adhere to treatment recommendations diligently.

Conclusion

The management of Chronic Myeloid Leukemia (CML) through diet is centered on the promotion of overall health, the improvement of treatment efficacy, and the reduction of adverse effects. Patients must consume a nutritious, well-balanced diet.

The immune system and overall cellular health can be supported by a high intake of fruits and vegetables, which provide vital vitamins, minerals, and antioxidants. Whole cereals provide essential fiber and energy, while lean proteins, including chicken, fish, lentils, and legumes, are essential for maintaining muscle mass and facilitating recovery.

Another essential element is hydration, which is essential for the prevention of treatment-related adverse effects and the preservation of bodily functions.

Adequate water consumption is essential for this purpose. Processed foods, sugary treats, and red meats should also be restricted by patients, as they can exacerbate inflammation and other health issues. It is strongly recommended that alcohol and tobacco be avoided, as they can exacerbate symptoms and impede treatment.

Individual health status, treatment plans, and adverse effects may all influence the specific nutritional requirements. Therefore, it is advisable to consult with healthcare providers, such as a dietitian, to adapt dietary choices to individual requirements. By adhering to these recommendations, patients with CML can more effectively manage their condition, improve their quality of life, and potentially enhance their treatment outcomes.

THE END